The
Resilient Mind
JOURNAL

Robert Armstrong
Library User Group

Here is a **clear, grounded, and empowering opening overview** for
☒ **Part 3 — Living Resilience**, written to naturally follow Parts 1 and 2 and set the tone for daily application.

Part 3 — Living Resilience

Resilience is not something you complete—it is something you live.

By the time you reach this section, you've done important inner work. You've learned to notice what you carry, understand your patterns, and strengthen your inner core with awareness and intention. *Living Resilience* is where that understanding becomes action—woven quietly into how you think, choose, relate, and respond each day.

This part of the journal focuses on practice rather than reflection alone. The pages ahead are designed to help you apply resilience in real situations: during stress, change, conflict, fatigue, and ordinary moments that once felt automatic. Here, resilience shows up in small decisions, calm pauses, healthy boundaries, and compassionate self-talk.

Living resilience does not mean staying strong all the time. It means knowing how to steady yourself when things feel unsteady, how to recover after setbacks, and how to care for your energy without guilt. It is about responding thoughtfully instead of reacting instinctively, and choosing progress that feels sustainable rather than forced.

As you move through this section, you may notice resilience becoming less effortful and more natural. It becomes part of how you listen, how you rest, how you communicate, and how you move forward—even when life remains unpredictable.

Take these pages slowly. Use them as daily check-ins, reflections after challenging moments, or quiet resets when needed. There is no finish line here—only a continued commitment to living with awareness, steadiness, and self-respect.

This is resilience in motion.

Ordering Information:
Quantity Sales: Special discounts are available for quantity purchases by corporations, assouciations, and others.
For details, contact the publisher at:
:Email: contact#libraryusergroup.com

For orders from U.S. trade bookstores and wholesalers, please contact contact your distribution channel.

———

The Resilient Mind Journal 3

———

ISBN: *978-1-63553-031-5*

Diaries & Journals

FIRST EDITION

Living With Intention

Write about how you want to show up in your life on purpose rather than by default.

_____

_____

_____

_____

_____

_____

_____

_____

_____

_____

_____

_____

_____

_____

How I Carry Resilience Forward

Reflect on ways resilience shows up in your everyday choices.

_____

_____

_____

_____

_____

_____

_____

_____

_____

_____

_____

_____

_____

_____

Responding to Challenges Today

Describe how you handled a recent challenge and what resilience looked like in that moment.

_____

_____

_____

_____

_____

_____

_____

_____

_____

_____

_____

_____

_____

_____

_____

_____

What Strength Looks Like in Practice
Write about how strength appears in your daily routines or interactions.

_____

_____

_____

_____

_____

_____

_____

_____

_____

_____

_____

_____

_____

_____

Staying Grounded Under Pressure
Reflect on what helps you stay steady when stress rises.

_____

_____

_____

_____

_____

_____

_____

_____

_____

_____

_____

_____

_____

Choosing Calm When I Can
Write about moments when choosing calm changed your experience.

_____

_____

_____

_____

_____

_____

_____

_____

_____

_____

_____

_____

_____

How I Recover After Hard Days
Describe what helps you reset after emotional or stressful days.

_____

_____

_____

_____

_____

_____

_____

_____

_____

_____

_____

_____

_____

_____

Resilience in Small Moments

Reflect on quiet acts of resilience you practice without noticing.

_____

_____

_____

_____

_____

_____

_____

_____

_____

_____

_____

_____

_____

_____

When I Meet Myself With Compassion
Write about how self-kindness supports your resilience.

_____

_____

_____

_____

_____

_____

_____

_____

_____

_____

_____

_____

_____

_____

Showing Up Even When It's Hard

Reflect on what motivates you to keep showing up.

_____

_____

_____

_____

_____

_____

_____

_____

_____

_____

_____

_____

_____

What Helps Me Stay Present

Write about habits or reminders that anchor you in the moment.

_____

_____

_____

_____

_____

_____

_____

_____

_____

_____

_____

_____

_____

_____

Navigating Change With Awareness

Reflect on how you handle change when it arises.

_____

_____

_____

_____

_____

_____

_____

_____

_____

_____

_____

_____

_____

_____

Resilience in My Relationships

Write about how resilience influences how you connect with others.

_____

_____

_____

_____

_____

_____

_____

_____

_____

_____

_____

_____

_____

_____

_____

How I Set Healthy Boundaries
Reflect on boundaries that protect your energy and well-being.

_____

_____

_____

_____

_____

_____

_____

_____

_____

_____

_____

_____

_____

Letting Go of What I Can't Control

Write about practicing acceptance in daily life.

_____

_____

_____

_____

_____

_____

_____

_____

_____

_____

_____

_____

_____

How I Handle Setbacks Now
Reflect on how your response to setbacks has evolved.

_____

_____

_____

_____

_____

_____

_____

_____

_____

_____

_____

_____

_____

Listening Before Reacting
Write about moments when pausing changed your response.

_____

_____

_____

_____

_____

_____

_____

_____

_____

_____

_____

_____

_____

_____

Choosing Progress Over Perfection
Reflect on how small steps build lasting strength.

_____

_____

_____

_____

_____

_____

_____

_____

_____

_____

_____

_____

_____

_____

How I Support Myself Through Stress
Write about supportive actions you take when stressed.

_____

_____

_____

_____

_____

_____

_____

_____

_____

_____

_____

_____

_____

_____

Resilience as a Daily Practice

Describe what resilience looks like on an ordinary day.

_____

_____

_____

_____

_____

_____

_____

_____

_____

_____

_____

_____

_____

_____

Finding Stability in Uncertainty
Reflect on how you remain steady when things feel unclear.

_____

_____

_____

_____

_____

_____

_____

_____

_____

_____

_____

_____

_____

_____

What Keeps Me Moving Forward
Write about motivations that help you persist.

_____

_____

_____

_____

_____

_____

_____

_____

_____

_____

_____

_____

_____

_____

_____

Trusting Myself in Decisions
Reflect on how self-trust strengthens resilience.

_____

_____

_____

_____

_____

_____

_____

_____

_____

_____

_____

_____

_____

_____

How I Adapt When Plans Change

Write about flexibility in action.

_____

_____

_____

_____

_____

_____

_____

_____

_____

_____

_____

_____

_____

Choosing Rest Without Guilt

Reflect on honoring rest as part of resilience.

_____

_____

_____

_____

_____

_____

_____

_____

_____

_____

_____

_____

_____

_____

How I Regulate My Emotions

Write about strategies that help you stay balanced.

_____

_____

_____

_____

_____

_____

_____

_____

_____

_____

_____

_____

_____

_____

Resilience in My Thoughts
Reflect on how you shape your thinking during challenges.

_____

_____

_____

_____

_____

_____

_____

_____

_____

_____

_____

_____

_____

_____

Practicing Patience in Real Life
Write about patience applied to daily situations.

_____

_____

_____

_____

_____

_____

_____

_____

_____

_____

_____

_____

_____

_____

How I Learn From Experience
Reflect on lessons gained through lived moments.

_____

_____

_____

_____

_____

_____

_____

_____

_____

_____

_____

_____

_____

Staying Kind Under Pressure
Write about choosing kindness toward yourself or others.

_____

_____

_____

_____

_____

_____

_____

_____

_____

_____

_____

_____

_____

How I Stay Connected to Myself
Reflect on practices that keep you aligned.

Resilience During Transitions

Write about navigating endings and beginnings.

_____

_____

_____

_____

_____

_____

_____

_____

_____

_____

_____

_____

_____

_____

Responding With Awareness
Reflect on moments you chose awareness over habit.

_____

_____

_____

_____

_____

_____

_____

_____

_____

_____

_____

_____

_____

_____

_____

How I Protect My Energy

Write about managing energy intentionally.

_____

_____

_____

_____

_____

_____

_____

_____

_____

_____

_____

_____

_____

_____

Resilience in Uncomfortable Moments
Reflect on staying steady through discomfort.

_____

_____

_____

_____

_____

_____

_____

_____

_____

_____

_____

_____

_____

_____

_____

Choosing Courage in Small Ways

Write about everyday courage.

_____

_____

_____

_____

_____

_____

_____

_____

_____

_____

_____

_____

_____

How I Handle Emotional Waves
Reflect on riding emotions without being overwhelmed.

_____

_____

_____

_____

_____

_____

_____

_____

_____

_____

_____

_____

_____

Practicing Self-Respect Daily
Write about honoring yourself through actions.

_____

_____

_____

_____

_____

_____

_____

_____

_____

_____

_____

_____

_____

How I Create Emotional Safety
Reflect on environments or behaviors that help you feel safe.

_____

_____

_____

_____

_____

_____

_____

_____

_____

_____

_____

_____

_____

_____

Resilience Without Resistance

Write about allowing life without constant struggle.

_____

_____

_____

_____

_____

_____

_____

_____

_____

_____

_____

_____

_____

_____

Staying Balanced When Life Is Busy
Reflect on maintaining equilibrium amid demands

_____

_____

_____

_____

_____

_____

_____

_____

_____

_____

_____

_____

_____

_____

How I Recenter When Off Track

Write about returning to your core.

_____

_____

_____

_____

_____

_____

_____

_____

_____

_____

_____

_____

_____

Choosing Awareness in Conversations

Reflect on mindful communication.

_____

_____

_____

_____

_____

_____

_____

_____

_____

_____

_____

_____

_____

Resilience in My Routines

Write about habits that support strength.

_____

_____

_____

_____

_____

_____

_____

_____

_____

_____

_____

_____

_____

_____

Handling Stress With Intention
Reflect on deliberate stress responses.

_____

_____

_____

_____

_____

_____

_____

_____

_____

_____

_____

_____

_____

_____

_____

_____

Trusting the Pace of My Life

Write about accepting timing.

_____

_____

_____

_____

_____

_____

_____

_____

_____

_____

_____

_____

_____

How I Handle Emotional Triggers

Reflect on responding rather than reacting.

_____

_____

_____

_____

_____

_____

_____

_____

_____

_____

_____

_____

_____

_____

Resilience in My Self-Talk

Write about speaking to yourself supportively.

_____

_____

_____

_____

_____

_____

_____

_____

_____

_____

_____

_____

_____

Staying Steady Through Uncertainty
Reflect on grounding strategies.

_____

_____

_____

_____

_____

_____

_____

_____

_____

_____

_____

_____

_____

_____

_____

How I Choose Calm Daily
Write about moments you consciously choose calm.

_____

_____

_____

_____

_____

_____

_____

_____

_____

_____

_____

_____

_____

_____

Living With Emotional Awareness

Reflect on noticing emotions as they arise.

_____

_____

_____

_____

_____

_____

_____

_____

_____

_____

_____

_____

_____

_____

How I Bounce Back Now

Write about recovery after difficulty.

_____

_____

_____

_____

_____

_____

_____

_____

_____

_____

_____

_____

_____

_____

Resilience in Decision-Making

Reflect on choosing with clarity.

_____

_____

_____

_____

_____

_____

_____

_____

_____

_____

_____

_____

_____

_____

How I Accept Imperfection in Practice
Write about letting things be unfinished.

_____

_____

_____

_____

_____

_____

_____

_____

_____

_____

_____

_____

_____

Navigating Challenges With Curiosity
Reflect on approaching difficulty with openness.

_____

_____

_____

_____

_____

_____

_____

_____

_____

_____

_____

_____

_____

_____

Resilience in My Body

Write about physical practices that support strength.

_____

_____

_____

_____

_____

_____

_____

_____

_____

_____

_____

_____

_____

_____

How I Stay Connected Under Stress

Reflect on maintaining connection.

_____

_____

_____

_____

_____

_____

_____

_____

_____

_____

_____

_____

_____

_____

_____

_____

Choosing Stability Over Chaos

Write about grounding choices.

_____

_____

_____

_____

_____

_____

_____

_____

_____

_____

_____

_____

_____

How I Handle Emotional Fatigue

Reflect on restoring energy.

_____

_____

_____

_____

_____

_____

_____

_____

_____

_____

_____

_____

_____

_____

Resilience as Consistency

Write about showing up repeatedly.

_____

_____

_____

_____

_____

_____

_____

_____

_____

_____

_____

_____

_____

Living With Self-Trust
Reflect on trusting your inner guidance.

_____

_____

_____

_____

_____

_____

_____

_____

_____

_____

_____

_____

_____

_____

_____

How I Respond to Disappointment

Write about meeting disappointment with care.

_____

_____

_____

_____

_____

_____

_____

_____

_____

_____

_____

_____

_____

_____

Resilience in Quiet Moments
Reflect on stillness as strength.

_____

_____

_____

_____

_____

_____

_____

_____

_____

_____

_____

_____

_____

_____

_____

_____

How I Balance Effort and Ease
Write about sustainable living.

_____

_____

_____

_____

_____

_____

_____

_____

_____

_____

_____

_____

_____

_____

Choosing Perspective Over Panic
Reflect on reframing challenges.

_____

_____

_____

_____

_____

_____

_____

_____

_____

_____

_____

_____

_____

_____

How I Stay Grounded in Conflict
Write about maintaining calm during tension.

_____

_____

_____

_____

_____

_____

_____

_____

_____

_____

_____

_____

_____

_____

Resilience in My Values

Reflect on living aligned with what matters.

_____

_____

_____

_____

_____

_____

_____

_____

_____

_____

_____

_____

_____

_____

How I Support My Future Self
Write about actions that help tomorrow.

_____

_____

_____

_____

_____

_____

_____

_____

_____

_____

_____

_____

_____

_____

Resilience in Everyday Choices

Reflect on daily decisions that build strength.

_____

_____

_____

_____

_____

_____

_____

_____

_____

_____

_____

_____

_____

_____

Living With Emotional Honesty

Write about authenticity in action.

_____

_____

_____

_____

_____

_____

_____

_____

_____

_____

_____

_____

How I Carry Lessons Forward
Reflect on applying what you've learned.

_____

_____

_____

_____

_____

_____

_____

_____

_____

_____

_____

_____

_____

Resilience When Things Feel Messy

Write about navigating imperfection.

_____

_____

_____

_____

_____

_____

_____

_____

_____

_____

_____

_____

_____

How I Stay Present During Stress
Reflect on grounding in real time.

_____

_____

_____

_____

_____

_____

_____

_____

_____

_____

_____

_____

_____

_____

Choosing Thoughtfulness Over Habit

Write about mindful action.

_____

_____

_____

_____

_____

_____

_____

_____

_____

_____

_____

_____

_____

_____

Resilience Through Self-Acceptance

Reflect on accepting yourself as you are.

_____

_____

_____

_____

_____

_____

_____

_____

_____

_____

_____

_____

_____

_____

How I Navigate Uncertainty With Care
Write about managing unknowns.

_____

_____

_____

_____

_____

_____

_____

_____

_____

_____

_____

_____

_____

_____

Resilience in My Daily Language

Reflect on words you choose.

_____

_____

_____

_____

_____

_____

_____

_____

_____

_____

_____

_____

_____

How I Create Stability for Myself

Write about self-support systems.

_____

_____

_____

_____

_____

_____

_____

_____

_____

_____

_____

_____

_____

_____

Living With Gentle Discipline

Reflect on structure without harshness.

_____

_____

_____

_____

_____

_____

_____

_____

_____

_____

_____

_____

_____

Resilience in Recovery

Write about bouncing back compassionately.

_____

_____

_____

_____

_____

_____

_____

_____

_____

_____

_____

_____

_____

_____

How I Meet Hard Moments Now
Reflect on present-day responses.

_____

_____

_____

_____

_____

_____

_____

_____

_____

_____

_____

_____

_____

_____

Choosing Alignment Over Approval

Write about living true to yourself.

_____

_____

_____

_____

_____

_____

_____

_____

_____

_____

_____

_____

_____

_____

Reflect on honoring boundaries.

_____

_____

_____

_____

_____

_____

_____

_____

_____

_____

_____

_____

_____

_____

How I Regain Balance Quickly

Write about returning to center.

_____

_____

_____

_____

_____

_____

_____

_____

_____

_____

_____

_____

_____

_____

Living With Emotional Flexibility

Reflect on adapting emotionally.

_____

_____

_____

_____

_____

_____

_____

_____

_____

_____

_____

_____

_____

_____

Resilience Through Self-Care

Write about caring for yourself intentionally.

_____

_____

_____

_____

_____

_____

_____

_____

_____

_____

_____

_____

_____

_____

_____

How I Sustain Strength Long-Term
Reflect on sustainable resilience.

_____

_____

_____

_____

_____

_____

_____

_____

_____

_____

_____

_____

_____

_____

Choosing Growth Without Pressure

Write about growing gently.

_____

_____

_____

_____

_____

_____

_____

_____

_____

_____

_____

_____

_____

_____

Resilience in Letting Things Be

Reflect on acceptance as strength.

How I Support Myself Daily

Write about ongoing self-support.

_____

_____

_____

_____

_____

_____

_____

_____

_____

_____

_____

_____

_____

As you come to the end of this section, take a moment to recognize how resilience has begun to live within you—not as something you force, but as something you practice with care. The pages you've written here reflect more than insight; they reflect choice, presence, and the willingness to meet life as it unfolds. Resilience will continue to grow through everyday moments—through pauses, boundaries, recovery, and compassion for yourself. You don't need to carry everything perfectly; you only need to keep returning to what steadies you. Let this be less of an ending and more of a continuation, knowing that resilience is now something you live, not just something you learn.

www.ingramcontent.com/pod-product-compliance
Lightning Source LLC
Chambersburg PA
CBHW011745020426
42333CB00022B/2721